How Your Brain Works

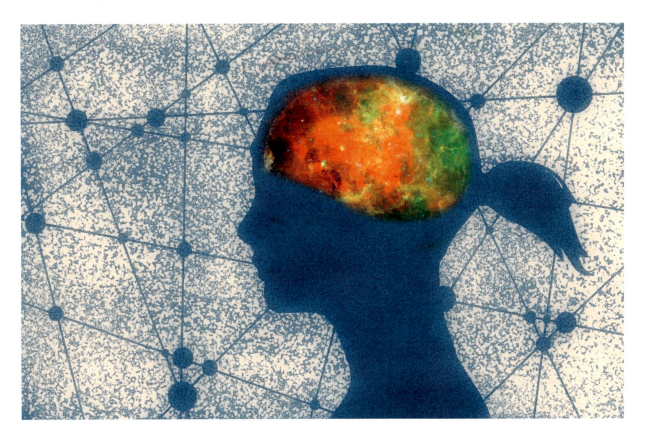

and How to Make It Work Smarter

by

Andrea Stehle, MdS

How Your Brain Works and How to Make It Work Smarter

Copyright 2018 by Andrea Stehle

First edition published August 2018

All rights reserved.

This book is protected under the copyright laws of the United States of America. It is intended for students, parents, and teachers in an educational setting. Any reproduction for profit or other unauthorized use of the material is prohibited.

Andrea Stehle is a Latin teacher at BASIS San Antonio Shavano Campus. She has been a teacher for 30 years and has conducted action research on metacognition with her students. She currently serves on the governing board of the American Classical League and is one of a hand full of researchers who has published articles on Latin vocabulary acquisition and retention in the 21st century.

Table of Contents

What is Metacognition? — page 1

How Does Your Brain Work? — page 4

    Make Learning an Active Verb — page 5

    Active Reading Strategies — page 8

What is Dual Encoding? — page 14

How Does Memory Work? — page 20

    Miller Study: The Limitations of Short-Term Memory — page 20

    Using Mnemonics — page 24

How Can Attitude Affect Learning? — page 26

    Smart Goals — page 27

Why Do I Run Out of Time? — page 29

    Steven Covey: Time Quadrants — page 33

    How Can a Planner Help Me? — page 35

    What is a Bullet Journal? — page 38

Metacognition and Studying — page 39

    Where Should I Study? — page 39

    What Should I Do Before I Study? — page 40

    Reflection After the Test — page 41

What is Knowledge Monitoring?	page 44
Flashcards	page 45
The Testing Effect	page 49
Is There More Than One Way to Be Smart?	page 51
Appendix:	
KMA	page 61
Steven Covey: Time Quadrants	page 65
Origin of Metacognition Highlighted	page 66
Stehle's Flashcard Data	page 67

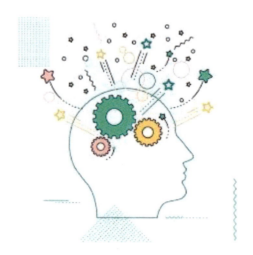

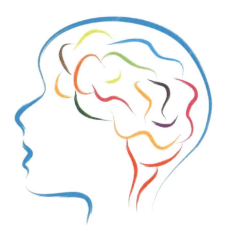

What is Metacognition?

When I was a little girl, my father used to tell me that school was a game. All I had to do was figure out the rules of the game and then play to win. For me the secret to success was participating in class, doing my homework, and asking questions. As long as I followed those rules I was good to go.

Of course, I had friends who did the same things I did, but without the same results. Some of my friends even spent more time studying than I did. ***Why did I make better grades?***

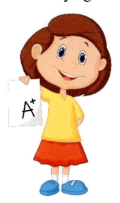

My friends, family, and teachers just assumed I was more successful because I was smarter than the other students. It wasn't until I got to college that I learned "smarter" was not the secret of my success.

While studying to become a teacher I discovered a concept that would have helped my friends do better in school. It is called **metacognition**. It is the brain's ability to understand and influence learning, ***and it is something everyone can do***.

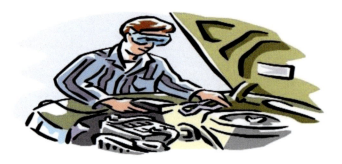

Just like the onboard computer in a car can monitor the engine and tell the mechanic where the trouble is, your brain can understand the learning process, reflect on how well it is working, and try new things that could make learning easier for you.

Learning is not magic. I did not make better grades in school because I was smarter than my friends. I was just better at seeing the "rules" of the game and understanding what to do to win. I was using metacognition, even before I knew what it was.

Metacognition may not be a skill everyone is born with, but it is a skill that everyone can learn and improve over time. The good news is that everyone has the potential to be the "smart" kid. The bad news is that no two people learn exactly the same way, so **you** are the only person who can discover how **your brain** works. The path to become a "smarter" learner is to tap into your personal metacognition and start using it to its full potential.

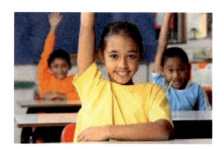

This is a guide book to metacognition. I will share with you what research has discovered about how the brain works, but that is only the beginning. The most important part of this guide book will involve exploring your individual learning styles and habits. The REFLECTIONS and TRY-IT exercises are ways for **you** to better understand **your brain** and develop **your metacognition**. The secret to success is simple – try out new ways of learning and see what works for you. Remember you are the only one who can walk the path and to tap into your metacognition.

It will require effort, but I promise you this. If you learn how your brain works, you can learn to make it work "smarter". That will be a win for you. Making your brain work smarter will help you in all your current classes in school, then it will help you in all your future classes, and finally as a lifelong learner. It will be worth your time and effort.

Thinking is the hardest work there is, which is probably the reason why so few engage in it.

Henry Ford

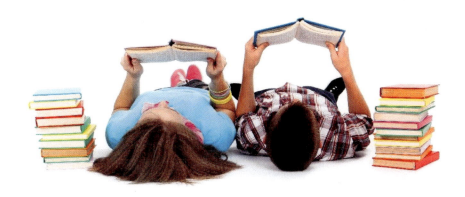

EVERY BRAIN IS DIFFERENT.

THERE ARE MANY DIFFERENT WAYS TO LEARN.

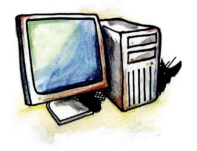

How does your brain work?

Think of your brain as a computer. Learning is just information processing. You must enter the new information into the computer and then save it. What you do to save new information is learning.

A quiz or test later is when you must retrieve the file you saved. You must be able to recall what you learned, or you didn't really learn it. How you process the new material (STUDY) will determine how easily you will be able to recall the material in the future?

The first thing to understand about learning and the **concept that can make the quickest improvement in your grades** is really very simple. Learning is not something that happens to you. Learning is something YOU do. Sitting in a classroom listening to a lecture or even reading a book for homework does not guarantee learning will take place. It is up to you to "process" the information. **Learning is an ACTIVE VERB.**

We have all been in a class where we let our mind wander and have no idea what the teacher said or reached the end of a page in a book and suddenly realized we had no clue what we had just read.

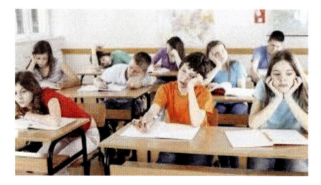

Such instances are examples of being human, but they are NOT examples of effective learning. Your brain must be engaged for learning to take place. Teachers try to make the lesson engaging, but in the end the burden for active learning falls on you the student.

HOW CAN YOU MAKE LEARNING AN ACTIVE VERB?

When you are listening to a teacher's lecture:

1) You should **focus** on what the teacher is explaining. Try to imagine it. Try to think of other examples. Try to participate in class discussions. Try to relate it to something you already know. Whatever works for you, just **think about it!**

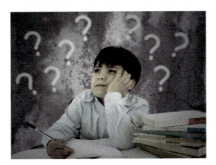

2) You should take **notes**. Often the teacher will have slides or write important things on the board. Copy anything your teacher emphasizes. Write down new vocabulary. Unless the teacher tells you to copy a definition word for word, try to put it in your own words. It is easier to learn things that way.

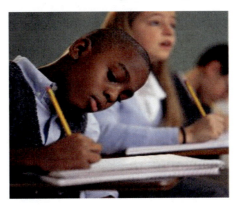

3) You should ask **questions**, and not just when you don't understand something. Ask questions when you want to know more. Ask questions about how a new idea connects with other things you have learned. Ask questions like "What if?" The more engaged your brain is in the topic, the easier learning becomes for you.

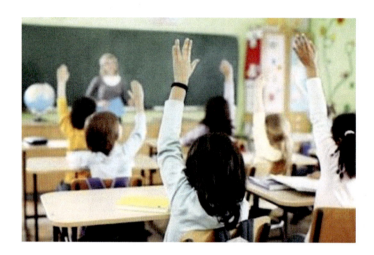

4) You should share your new knowledge with others. Research shows that "**teaching**" is the most effective way to learn. You can tell someone else (Mom, Dad, a sibling, or a friend) what the teacher's lecture taught you. ***Spend five minutes in the evening talking about what you learned in school that day.*** This simple addition to your nightly homework routine will help you process new information and help you remember it for quizzes and tests.

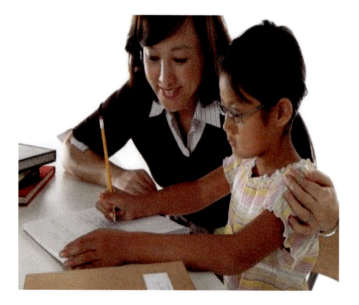

REFLECTION

Reread the suggestions for making a teacher's lecture a more ACTIVE learning process. Have you tried one of them? Did it make the new material easier to remember? How did you do on the quiz/test?

_____
_____
_____
_____
_____
_____
_____
_____
_____
_____

TRY-IT

Ask your parents to read suggestion #4.

Try making it a nightly routine for them to ask what you learned today, and then spend five minutes every night "teaching" your parents.

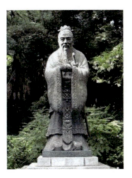

I hear and I forget.
I see and I remember.
I do and I understand.
Confucius

ACTIVE Reading Strategies

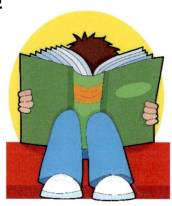

1) You should read in **small chunks** (no more than 1-3 pages at a time). Stop and "think about" what you have read before you move on to the next small chunk. Your brain needs time to process the new information.

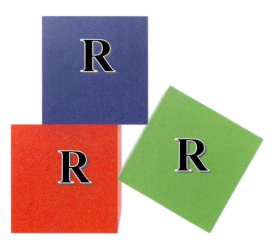

2) You should spend a little time making sure you understand what you are reading. There is an ACTIVE reading strategy known as the **3R Method**. I teach it to college freshmen, but I recommend it for AP students as well.

The three R's stand for **Read, Recite,** and **Reread**. Here is how it works. When you finish reading a section of the textbook, close the book and try to recite (or even better try to write down) what you just read in your own words. If there are gaps in your understanding, go back and reread that part of the text.

3) You should take **notes** while reading. Use section headings in the textbook to help outline what you read. Copy new vocabulary and define them in your own words. Make lists of important concepts and topics.

Here is an example of notes over what you just read in this book.

<u>Four ways to make learning Active</u>   p. 5 & 6

1) Focus on what the teacher is saying. Think about it.
2) Take notes during lecture. Write new words and definitions.
3) Ask questions. Engage your brain.
4) Share learning with others. Teach what you learn.

4) You should **highlight** important vocabulary and concepts on your papers and in your textbook (when you are allowed to). This is a way of processing the information. Later, rereading a highlighted text is a useful way to review for quizzes and tests.

A tip for highlighting with the main ideas and important text already highlighted.

Research suggests that ==students who highlight important details when they read have higher levels of comprehension and retention==. This is good news for students who can use this active reading strategy to decide what is important and focus in on what to study for quizzes and tests.

Be careful though. ==You can't highlight just anything==. You must highlight the main ideas and definitions. To do that correctly takes time. Here is what I recommend. ==You should read the text first – no highlighting.== On the ==second reading you should highlight the main ideas or new words and their definitions.== Highlight only the important words, phrases and sentences.

••

TRY-IT

Use the 3R Reading Method on a reading assignment for one of your classes.

READ 1-3 PAGES OF THE TEXTBOOK.

CLOSE THE BOOK.

NOW WRITE DOWN THE IMPORTANT DETAILS OF WHAT YOU READ   (AS MUCH AS YOU CAN REMEMBER).

_____
_____
_____
_____
_____
_____
_____
_____
_____
_____
_____
_____

NOW OPEN UP THE BOOK.

REREAD and COMPLETE NOTES.

REFLECTION

Do you feel the 3R Method helped you understand what you read? Do you think it will help you remember the material for the quiz/test? WHY?

_____
_____
_____
_____
_____
_____
_____

Return to this REFLECTION after the Quiz or Test? How did you do? Did the 3R Reading Method help? Did you use the notes to study? Will you use this method again? Why?

_____
_____
_____
_____
_____

Reading is Fun!

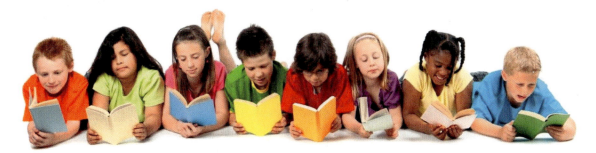

TRY-IT

This is a passage from a paper on Metacognition.

1) Read it.
2) Then read it again and highlight the main ideas.
3) Compare your highlights with the highlighted passage in the appendix.

The Origins of Metacognition

The term metacognition began with an American developmental psychologist named John H. Flavell. Educational researchers had been studying smart students (the ones that were more successful in school) and trying to define what characteristics and skills made them smarter than their peers. Flavell and others found that smart students often did better than their peers in multiple subjects. How could they be better in math, science, reading, and history? They couldn't all have stronger background knowledge or more interest in every subject. Some other factor had to be at work.

It turned out that most smart students did have one thing in common. They were all good at learning new things. They could explain how they learned, learn from their mistakes, and knew what study methods worked best for them. They thought about learning. Researchers had discovered what made some students smarter than others and thus was born the science of metacognition.

Flavell defined metacognition as knowledge about and control of one's thinking. Metacognition is a process. For example, a person who is engaging in metacognition notices that they are having more trouble learning Biology than learning English. They think about the similarities and differences in their approaches to learning those two subjects and decide what factors might be making Biology harder. A metacognitive thinker then systematically experiments with new ways to study Biology. They don't stop trying out new ways to learn until they find the ones that help them understand and remember Biology most effectively.

Metacognition can be as important to the learning process as the content of the subject. Novice learners spend all their time and effort studying with little planning or reflection. Sometimes they are successful and sometimes they are not. To be a metacognitive learner, students think about and plan for studying. How else can they be sure they spend enough time and study the right material. After they get back their grade on the quiz or test, a metacognitive learner will reflect on how well their studying worked and how it might be improved in the future. To truly use and improve metacognition a student must not just understand how their brain works but continually monitor and adjust their efforts to maximize learning.

TRY-IT again

Answer these questions *without looking back at the passage*, then use the passage to check your answers.

Which researcher first used the term metacognition? _____

What did researchers find smart students had in common?

_____
_____
_____
_____

Define metacognition.

_____

What do metacognitive learners do BEFORE they study?

_____
_____
_____
_____

What do metacognitive learners do AFTER the quiz or test?

_____
_____
_____
_____

What is Dual Encoding?

Memory in our brain works a little like books on the shelves of a library. Every new experience and learning opportunity is a different book. You are constantly adding new books to your library.

If you want to find a specific book, you must be able to find the shelf you put it on. That can be hard. Libraries are huge places full of many books (memories). It is easy for things to get lost.

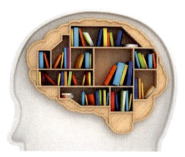

Neuroscientists have explored the biochemistry of memory. When the brain learns something new, a chemical pathway is created to that specific piece of knowledge. The neurons in your brain are permanently changed by the information or memory. The scientists call the process ENCODING. When we want to "remember" the information, our brain must follow the same chemical pathway to find it again.

Being able to remember what you learned is vital to success in school, but it is not always easy. Have you ever lost a file on a computer because you could not remember what you called it?

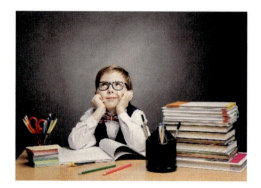

That feeling that the word you are trying to remember is on the tip of your tongue is your brain trying to find the pathway back to where the word is encoded.

Have you ever studied and thought you were ready, but then could not remember the information for the test? You may have had the information in your brain. The problem is you could not find it.

Now imagine that you purposefully learned the word or concept two different ways. **Your brain would create two different pathways to the same information. That would double your chances of finding the right pathway and remembering.** That will make your life easier when it comes time to take the test or quiz.

This is a metacognitive concept is called **Dual Encoding**.

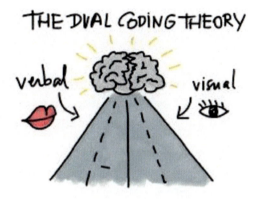

There are many ways to encoding information into the brain. Dual Encoding Theory says we should always choose two.

Read it.	Write it.
Recite it.	Draw it.
Explain it.	Listen to it.
Sing it.	See it.
Act it out.	Practice it.

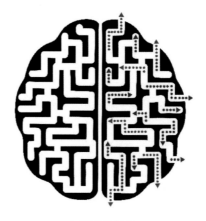

REFLECTION

Sometimes a song will remind you of someone you hadn't thought about in a long time, or a smell will make you remember something that happened in the past that you hadn't thought about in years. Explain how these are examples of Dual Encoding.

_____
_____
_____
_____
_____

TRY-IT

Next time you must learn new vocabulary for a class, try studying the words TWO different ways. I recommend you use the study method you are most comfortable with, but then study the words again using an encoding method that is NEW to you.

Over the next few weeks you should try out ALL the different encoding methods and see which ones work best for you. Improving your metacognition requires you to tryout new study methods and decide which ones you will keep using.

Helpful Hints:

Some students are reluctant to try out NEW encoding methods, because they aren't sure they will work for them. They may not, but you never know until you try.

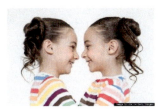

Remember no two brains learn in exactly the same way. Everyone has different strengths and talents. Metacognitive Theory says you should explore all the different study methods and then use what works BEST for your brain.

If you are an artist, then drawing pictures of what you are learning plays right into your natural talent. If you are an athlete, then try moving around while you study.

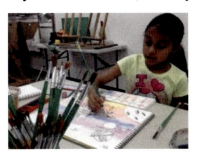 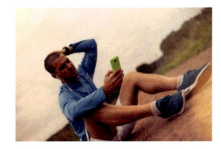

If you like to sing, then sing what you want to learn. (That is how you learned your ABC's, isn't it?)

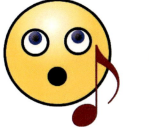 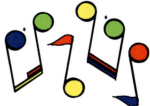

Many students will record their notes and listen to them to study. My own daughter likes to listen to the book while she reads her novels for English class. By using two encoding methods at the same time she improves her reading comprehension and her grades on the quiz.

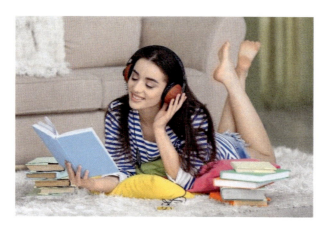

Look for FREE audio books on YouTube for most popular readings assignments.

Next time someone says they don't understand how to do something and asks you for the answer, ***don't give it to them***. Instead you should ***explain how you figured it*** out and guide them to the correct answer. That way you benefit even more than they do, because you have just encoded the information in a whole new way.

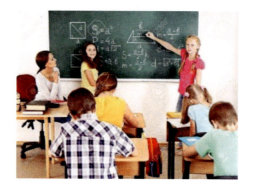

Did I mention that TEACHING is the best method for learning?

Research says that students tend to remember

    10% of what they READ

    20% of what they HEAR

    30% of what they SEE

    50% of what they SEE and HEAR

    70% of what they SAY

    90% of what they SAY and DO

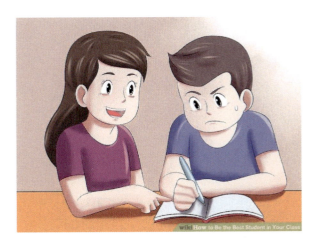

(Saying and doing! That is TEACHING.)

How Does Memory Work?

After you see or hear something, your mind holds the experience in short term memory. This sensory input in short term memory can be a new vocabulary word you just heard to your teacher say or the color of a flower you just spotted in the garden. Whatever the type of experience, sensory input in short term memory is limited. If you don't use it, you will lose it. In fact, information in short term memory only lasts 20 to 30 seconds before we "forget" it.

To remember something we have seen or heard longer than 30 seconds, the sensory input must be transferred to long term memory. This process from short term memory to long term memory is accomplished through focus and repetition. By recalling the thought and replaying it in our mind, we actually change the chemistry of the neurons in the brain and create a pathway to that information.

Miller Study: The limitations of Short-term Memory

In 1956 George Miller of Harvard University conducted a study which demonstrated the normal capacity of short term memory. The TRY-IT below replicates this experiment.

TRY-IT

Below is a list of words. Look at the list for 1 minute. Then turn the page and follow the instructions. (Don't look ahead!)

CAT	FLOWER	FIREMAN	BUS
PONY	TOASTER	MICROPHONE	ICE CREAM
POTATO	SUN	LEAF	TROPHY
DESK	TRAIN	SQUIRREL	TEACHER

Now write down as many of the words as you can remember.
      (Don't cheat by looking back.)

potato	desk
toaster	teacher
sun	squirrel
train	bee
pony	cat

How many could you remember? __10__

Miller's 1956 study found that most people can remember 7 words (plus or minus 2). That would be somewhere between five and nine words. What does this mean for you?

First, trying to memorize things at the last minute only engages your short term memory, so you can only remember 5-9 answers. That may not be enough to do very well on the test/quiz. Second, finding ways to process information from our short term memory into long term memory would increase our ability to remember it later for things like the Final Exams and AP Tests.

Fortunately, Miller himself suggested a solution. He said that by organizing the stimulus input into smaller groupings, we manage to break (or at least stretch) the informational bottleneck of short term memory.

Reflection

Have you ever wondered why telephone numbers work the way they do? How do they use Miller's findings?

___
___
___

TRY-IT again

The good news is you are not limited to 5-9 answers. There is a memorization technique called **chunking** that could help you improve the number of words you can recall in the Miller experiment. Let's try it.

Look at the list again. Look for words that having something in common. For instance, cat, pony & squirrel are all animals. Try to do this for as many of the words on the list as possible. This process is called **chunking**.

Spend three minutes chunking the words on the list before you turn to the next page. (You may rewrite parts of the lists and make notes of chunking below.)

CAT	FLOWER	FIREMAN	BUS
PONY	TOASTER	MICROPHONE	ICE CREAM
POTATO	SUN	LEAF	TROPHY
DESK	TRAIN	SQUIRREL	TEACHER

Try to write down as many of the words as you can remember. (Don't cheat by looking back.)

cat	flower
fireman	bus
pony	toaster
microphone	ice cream
sun	potato
leaf	trophy
train	desk
squirrel	teacher

How many could you remember this time? __16__

Reflection:

Most people are able to remember more words the second time. Do you think it was the chunking or could there be other reasons?

_____
_____
_____
_____
_____
_____
_____
_____

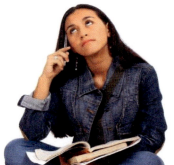

     If you mentioned that it was the second time you studied the same list or that you spent more time thinking about and processing the words when you were chunking, then you are using your metacognition. You are starting to think about your learning and discover how **your brain** works.

How to Use Mnemonics

There is another study method that makes use of the idea of chunking. Mnemonics are memory tools. They help find the pathway to larger chunks of information by providing clues to help you retrieve the information.

One type of mnemonic is creating a WORD from the first letter of each word in a list. It helps you remember all the words in the list. This type of mnemonic is called an **acronym**. You have probably already used this one in school.

FANBOYS   the seven coordinating conjunctions

for   and   nor   but   or   yet   so

IPMAT   the phases of mitosis.

interphase   prophase   metaphase   anaphase   telophase

HOMES   the five Great Lakes.

Huron   Ontario   Michigan   Erie   Superior

PAIN   first declension words that are masculine in Latin.

Poeta   Agricola   Incola   Nauta

Another type of mnemonic is the SENTENCE. Again you use the first letter of each word to create a crazy sentence that is intended to provide a retrieval clue to help you remember the information in a specific order. These are also popular in school.

My Dear Aunt Sally is intended to help you remember the order of operation in math. They are multiplication, division, addition and then subtraction.

King **P**hillip **C**ame **O**ver **F**or **G**ood **S**oup is the order of taxonomy in Biology, which is Kingdom, Phylum, Class, Order, Family, Genus, Species.

Every **G**ood **B**oy **D**oes **F**ine stands for the names of the notes on the lines of the treble staff.

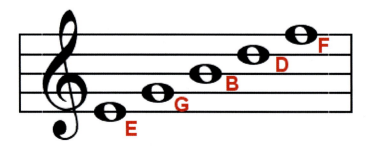

I cannot stress enough the power of mnemonics in improving memory capacity. *Ask any doctor how they got through medical school.* It was the first metacognitive tool I learned. When I was a junior in high school, I took Anatomy and Physiology. I found it challenging. The last six weeks we were required to identify the names of bones, muscles, organs, and nerves during dissections. It was the hardest part of the class. My lab partner was the Valedictorian of the Senior class who showed me how to create mnemonics to help memorize all those names and locations. It made the learning easy. To everyone's amazement, including my own, I made a 100 that six weeks.

TRY IT

Find a list (characteristics, steps, etc) that you need to memorize for a class. Create your own mnemonic. (acronym or sentence)

How Can Attitude Affect Learning?

As a teacher I have heard too many students say, "The teacher gave me a bad grade on the test." or "I passed the quiz without studying." Both of these statements clearly show that the students are not using metacognition. In fact, both statements show that these students aren't taking responsibility for their learning and therefore cannot hope to improve.

The teacher gave me a bad grade. Don't fall into this trap. The teacher does not give a student a grade. The student earns a failing grade. If you don't REFLECT on the failure, then you are doomed to repeat it. Look at how you studied, when you studied, what you studied, and figure out where you went wrong. If you don't know what you did wrong or how to do better next time, go to your teacher's tutoring. That is what it is there for.

I passed without studying. This trap is even worse. Don't get cocky. Either you already knew the material, or you actively participated in class and did all your homework. Give yourself CREDIT. You didn't need to a separate study session because you were ready for the test. A good metacognitive student will know what they know and not waste time with unnecessary studying. *I knew the material so well that I didn't have to spend extra time studying for the test* – that is metacognition.

REFLECTION

Sometimes you didn't study and don't know the material but make a lucky guess on the quiz or test. Will you be ready to use this information later in the course? Will you know it for the midterm or final exam? Why? What should you do?

_____
_____
_____
_____
_____
_____
_____

ATTITUDE CAN BE MORE IMPORTANT THAN APTITUDE.

Smart goals

IF YOU DON'T KNOW WHERE YOU ARE GOING, THEN YOU ARE GOING NOWHERE.

This bit of wisdom is something everyone would do well to remember. Even if you don't realize it, everyone is motivated by goals. *I want to graduate from high school. I want to get a good job.* These are long term goals and they are what motivate us to keep trying in school. A goal is what helped me get through Hemingway's **Old Man and the Sea**. I didn't really enjoy the book, but I made myself finish reading it, so I could write the paper on it to pass English II and eventually graduate from high school.

It is possible to use short term GOALS to help you on a daily basis. Short term goals are the steps we need to take to reach our big goals – like graduation. Think of it them as a checklist that keeps you on track and can help keep you motivated. You want the goals to be SMART. (specific, measurable, achievable, realistic and time-based) Here are some examples of SMART goals.

1) I will study in three different fifteen-minute sessions to prepare for the Biology Quiz on Friday.
2) I will finish the rough draft of my English essay before dinner and give it to my older brother to review.
3) I will make and use flashcards to study for my Latin vocabulary quiz next week.

Notice that these goals were specific and measurable. They didn't include grades, but instead were focused on activities intended to improve academic performance. They were time-based, because when they had to be done was included in the goal.

Because they are specific, it will be easy to determine if the goal has been reached. It is also important to reward yourself for reaching short term goals. Celebrating success with a candy bar, the next episode of your favorite TV show, or time spent texting your friends will produce positive feelings and motivate you in the future.

Similarly, if you fail to reach a goal, you need to reflect on what went wrong and how you could do better next time. A metacognitive learner is always looking out for new ways to improve their thinking. They never let failure stop them, but see it as an opportunity to learn and grow.

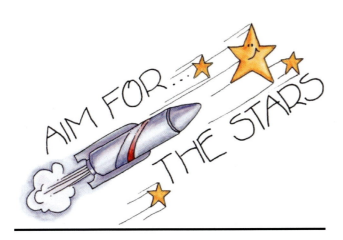

My favorite Latin quote is *Ad Astra Per Aspera*. It means "To the stars through hard work."

It is important to note that goals must be achievable and realistic, but challenging enough to help us improve and grow. Research shows that goals that challenge us to reach just a little higher than we think we can are the most effective. They make you push yourself, increase your satisfaction with school, and improve your self-confidence for the future. Warning: Don't make the goal too lofty. If you set a goal that you could never possibly reach, then you are setting yourself up for failure. Success comes in steps, not a giant leap to the finish line.

TRY IT

Think about the steps you need to take to improve your metacognitive thinking. Write a SMART goal for yourself. Remember it must be specific, measurable, achievable, realistic and time-based.

_____
_____
_____
_____

Reflection

Did you reach your goal? Why? _____
_____
_____

<u>Why Do I Run Out of Time?</u>

There are many people and activities competing for your time and attention when you get home from school. Your English teacher wants you to read, your math teacher wants you to do problems, your Mom wants you to take out the trash, your friends want to text them back and your little brother wants you to play on the X-box with him. You can't do it all at the same time, and if you don't do them in the right order you may not be able to get them all done.

This is a demo I do for my classes to illustrate how Time Management works.

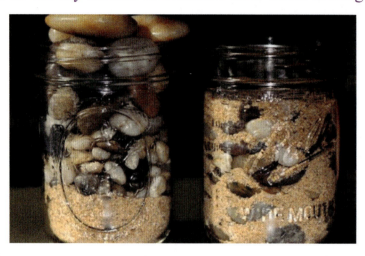

You are given a large empty jar. Beside it are three large rocks, a bunch of pebbles, and a cup of sand. Your task it to fit them all into the jar.

If you start with the sand, then add the pebbles, they fill up most of the jar and you can't fit in all three of the big rocks.

If you start with the three big rocks, they take up much of the jar, but with a difference. There are small pockets of space between the big rocks and the glass, so when you add the pebbles they fall down into the empty space. Even though it looked like they wouldn't fit, they did. Now pour the cup of sand into the jar. It falls down into the space between the pebbles. THIS WAY everything fits in the jar.

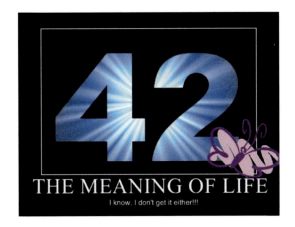

If you didn't get the joke, I highly recommend reading the book.

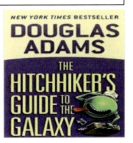

Reflection: What does it all mean?

Which item in the demo represents the major/important things in your life?

_____

Which item in the demo represents all the small daily tasks you must do?

_____

Which item in the demo represents all your fun activities and free time?

_____

What do you think the jar represents?

_____

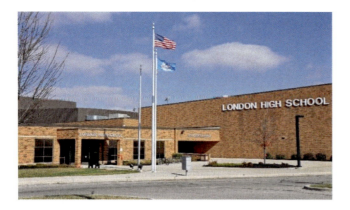

The major/important things in your life are the **big rocks**. Most people only have 2-3 big things each day. Go to school. Study for a test. Work on a project.

Remember that major/important things don't have to take up all your time. They just have to be the things that you get done FIRST.

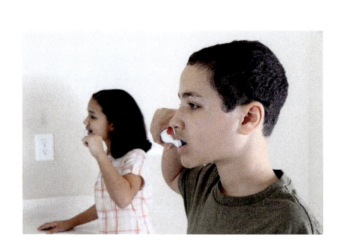 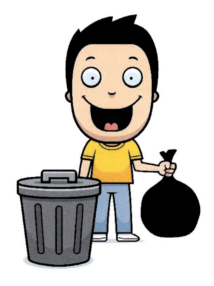

The **pebbles** were the small daily tasks you must do. Brush your teeth. Take out the trash. Clean your room. Do your homework. You have to make time to get them done.

Homework is a pebble? Yes! Smaller reading, writing, and math assignments that you have to do everyday should have their own regularly scheduled time and place. Make them a habit, just like taking bath or eating dinner.

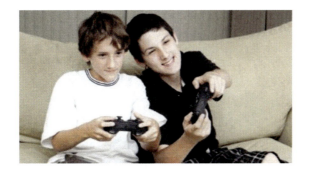

The **sand** is all the things in life you want to do for fun. Watching TV. Playing video games. Texting your friends. Just sitting in the back yard staring up at the sky.

Remember ***that you don't have to give up the fun stuff***, but <mark>you have to take care of the big rocks and pebbles first</mark>. There is plenty of time as long as you prioritize.

HELPFUL HINT: Mixing It Up

When studying for a test or working through the steps of a major project, it is easy to lose focus. What should have taken an hour to complete drags into two hours because your mind wanders, or you get distracted. **This is not the most effective use of your time.**

Try spending 20 minutes studying. It will be easier to stay focused for such a short period of time. Don't let yourself get distracted. When the 20 minutes are up, give yourself a 10 minute break to do something fun. (I suggest you set a timer on your phone to make sure you stick to your timetable.)

After your 10 minutes break, go back for another 20 minutes of studying. You can do this with homework, too. Our brains work harder when they concentrate for short periods of time, knowing they have a fun activity waiting when they are done.

TIME QUADRANTS

Sean Covey wrote a book called "**The 7 Habits of Highly Successful Teens**". *It is a book all teens should read.* One of his most valuable lessons talks about putting first things first. There are things in our life that are urgent and other things we have plenty of time to do. There are also things in our life that are important and other things that are not so important to our success. Covey says how and when we take care of the tasks in our life can be divided into four categories. To see why he calls them TIME QUADRANTS check out the graph in the appendix.

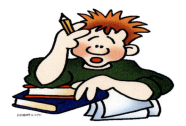

The first type is the **Procrastinator**. This person doesn't work on the important things until they become urgent. It is not that they don't know the project is due on Friday; it is just that they keep putting off getting started, because they have plenty of time. They are the ones who stay up all night to finish a paper or cram for the test at the last minute. They create their own crisis and stress, because they put off getting to work until the deadline is looming.

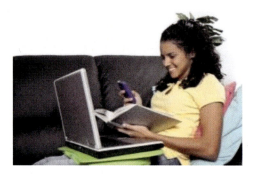

The second type is the Yes-Man. This person doesn't get the important things in their life done, because they are too busy doing what everyone else wants them to do. They are the ones who don't get much studying done, because they keep answering text messages. They let less important things take over their lives and run out of time for their big rocks. This person lets other people's problems and peer pressure keep them from what they need to do to be successful.

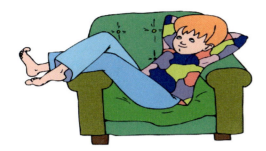

    The third type is the **Slacker**. This is the person who take fun activities to excess. They don't just watch TV; they bing watch the entire season in one sitting. They play video games until past midnight and then sleep until noon more days than they don't. They have never had a job, because they never actually tried to find one. In school they are the student who never gets around to doing their part of the group project or remembering to return the book they borrowed from you.

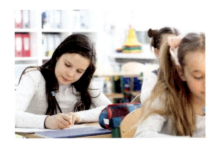

    The fourth type is the **Prioritizer**. This is a person who looks at all the things they have to do and want to do and decides what is most important and most urgent. They put important things first and plan ahead. They are the person who starts working on the project the day the teacher assigns it. They begin studying for a test days in advance. They have plenty of time for family, friends and fun, because they are not cramming for quizzes or struggling to finish the paper for English due the next day. They have a balance to their life and fit their big rocks, pebbles, and sand into the jar.

REFLECTION

Which Time Quadrant sounds most like a metacognitive student? Why?

_____
_____
_____
_____
_____
_____

How Can a Planner Help Me?

School is a full-time job. It can get hectic. You have many different classes with different homework assignments, different quizzes/tests to study for, and different projects to be working on. Even the best student cannot remember all the due dates and deadlines without a little help. If you don't want to get in trouble for forgetting to do something, the solution is simple. WRITE IT DOWN.

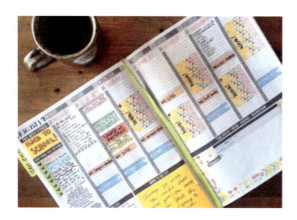

Reflection

Ask your parents or other adults whether they use a planner/calendar to keep track of doctor's appointments, deadlines at work, school functions, etc. How will learning to "plan" in school help you later in life?

_____
_____
_____
_____
_____
_____

Getting a planner or calendar is a good beginning, but it is how you use it that will improve your time management and academic performance. Many schools and teachers require students to have a planner. Here are some suggestions for making the most out of it.

RULES for KEEPING a PLANNER

1) Write in your planner for every class, every day. You need to be consistent and make it a habit.

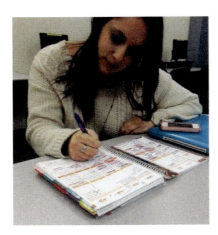

2) Write in your planner as soon as the teacher announces homework, quizzes, tests or project due dates. Don't wait or you may forget to write it down or remember the wrong date.

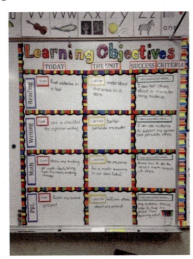

3) Look at your planner every night. What is due tomorrow? What is due two days from now? Do you have a quiz/test that you need to study for or a project to be working on?

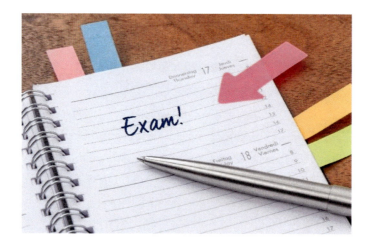

Helpful Hint:

Color coding a planner can make it easier to see what is important at a glance. You can put all TEST dates in one color and all homework in another. Some students color code by class to make it easier to see what they have to do in each subject. Remember there is no wrong way to do it. Try out different color coding systems until you find the one that works for you.

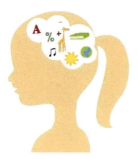

WE HAVE TOO MANY THINGS TO REMEMBER WITHOUT A LITTLE HELP.

What is a bullet journal?

Bullet journals are an alternate form of planner. The only thing you truly need to start a bullet journal is a blank notebook or journal and a pen. Bullet journals give the owner the power to create their own planner and make it fit your lifestyle. You have the creative freedom to design and create that regular planners lack.

Minimalist bullet journals are as basic and simple as you can get. They are designed for those who are very busy or people who are not artistically inclined.

Advanced bullet journals contain extravagant layouts and images that allow more creative owners to express themselves. This journal allows the owner to exercise their creativity and tryout new ideas and drawings.

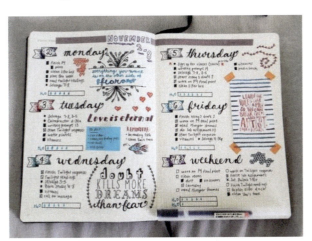
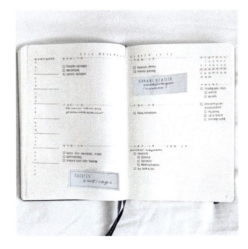

My daughter Amanda uses a bullet journal to track habits, make to-do lists, keep records of progress towards goals, plus all the things a normal planner would have.

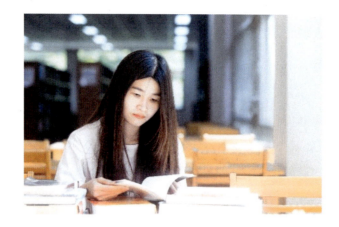

Metacognition and Studying

Where Should I Study?

Homework and studying will be something you do almost every night. You need to find a place that works for you. Here are some suggestions when looking for the perfect spot:

1) It should be a **comfortable space**. It should have good lighting; not be too hot or too cold; have a nice place to sit and plenty of room to spread out and work.

2) It should be a **free from distractions**. Trying to do homework in the same room where your little brother is playing video games is NOT going to help you stay focused. Your bedroom may or may not be the perfect spot. You will have to decide. You need to be able to get things done.

3) It should have the **supplies you need** to work. Paper, pens, map pencils, eraser, computer, textbook, etc. You should have space to store your "study stuff" while you are not using it.

4) It should be a **space you can use anytime**. You need to get into a study routine – having specific times when you work on homework and study. Your space should be available and distraction free when you need to work. (For example: Trying to study at the kitchen table while your Mom is trying to make dinner may not be the best choice.)

What Should I Do Before Studying?

Remember that a metacognitive learner does not start studying until they have planned what they will do. To work smarter, it is important to decide when, where, and how you will study. The previous section discussed finding the right spot to study. The section before that discussed using your planner to make sure you find enough time to study. Now it is time to decide how you will study.

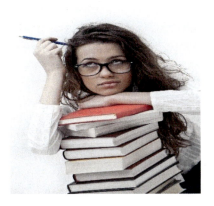

One important thing research tells us about studying is that those really long study sessions the night before the test aren't the most efficient or effective way to learn. Although it might seem like devoting two hours the night before will make you do well on the test, the reality is your brain can only take in so much new information in one sitting. You are wasting your time and effort rereading notes or textbooks after more than about 45 minutes. If your brain is tired and losing focus, no learning is taking place.

The smarter method is to study a little bit at a time over several days. Most of the time the teacher gives you notice about an upcoming quiz or test. If you have several days until the test, you have several days to study. Don't wait to get started.

1) You should plan two 15-20 minute study sessions for each day you have until the test. Studying multiple days will help you remember the material better.

2) Divide up the material you need to learn. Don't try to cover everything each study session. Reviewing what you learned last time and then moving on to new material is best.

3) Try different encoding methods during different study sessions. Remember you want to Dual Encode everything you learn to give you twice the chance to recall it for the quiz/test.

REFLECTION AFTER THE TEST

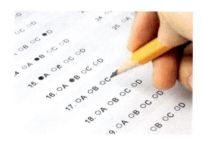

When you get back your graded test or quiz, ***don't throw it away***! You may have heard the phrase "learning from your mistakes". That is the goal. There is a lot a metacognitive learner can gain by reviewing the exam. Reread the questions you missed. Correct your mistakes and use notes/textbook to find the right answers. If you have any doubts or concerns about a question, ASK YOUR TEACHER.

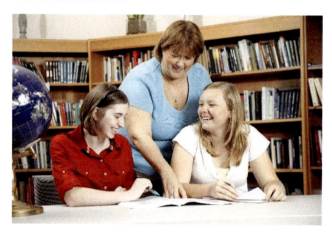

Many teachers offer extra points for doing corrections or going over a test in tutoring. **Take advantage of this opportunity.** It will improve your grade in the present and help you do better on future assessments. <u>The test is NOT the end of the learning process</u>. Understanding concepts from one chapter may be required to do the lessons in the next chapter. In many cases the concepts and questions on your test will be covered again by midterms and final exams.

Don't just go over the questions you missed. Also look at the questions you got correct. Reflect on what you did well and celebrate your strengths. How did you study for the questions you got correct? How much time did you spend on those concepts? Decide which parts of your study routine worked and consider how you might improve your study habits for the next test.

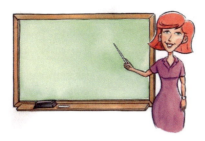

Try to think like the teacher. When you are studying, try to imagine what you would ask, if you were the teacher. **Take advantage of test reviews**. Teachers will often give you hints about what will be on the test, what material you should concentrate on, and the format the questions will be asked. If they keep saying the same thing or covering the same idea, THAT IS IMPORTANT.

TRY-IT

After you get back your next major test, try one of these metacognitive approaches.

1) Did I study the right things?

Reread the questions on the test. Where did the teacher get each question? Was it from the textbook or from lecture notes? Was it something the teacher talked about in class or had you practice as homework?

Helpful Hint: Did some ideas appear more than once? Was the definition in the textbook and the teacher's lecture? Were there homework assignments that practiced something you learned in class? If any topic or definition comes up more than once, IT IS IMPORTANT. Study it.

2) Did I study the right way?

Reread the questions on the test. Mark the way(s) you encoded or studied for each question. Is there a pattern? Which study method(s) produced the most correct answers? Which study method(s) had the most missed questions? How could you improve your studying for the next test?

Helpful hint: Go over tests and quizzes where you tried a new study method or used Dual Encoding and decide if these methods worked for you. Remember every brain is different and only you can determine what works best for you.

3) Did I study long enough?

How many study sessions did you have for this test? Over how many days? Was it enough? Could you have done better if you had spent more time studying? Look at your planner. Was there extra time you could have used to study?

Helpful hint: Studying for tests and quizzes is a marathon not a sprint. You must find time for multiple short study sessions. Keep increasing the number of study sessions until you discover how much time your brain needs to prepare. It won't be the same for every student.

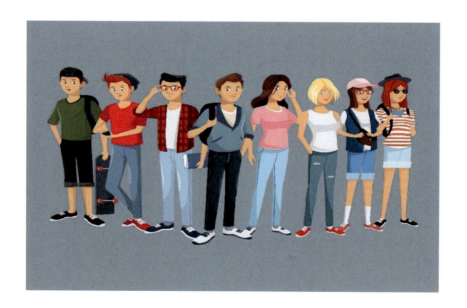

What is Knowledge Monitoring?

One of the most important discoveries made while doing research on metacognition is that not everyone can accurately judge what they do and don't know. The concept is called Knowledge Monitoring. There is a Knowledge Monitoring Assessment in the appendix of this book, if you would like to find out how accurate your knowledge monitoring skills are.

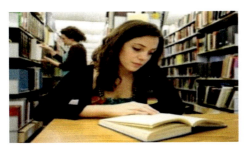

Students who are good knowledge monitors have a major advantage over students who are not. Poor knowledge monitors may waste time studying things they already know or stop studying too soon thinking they know the material when they don't. Your brain is not doing it on purpose. Knowledge Monitoring is simply a skill some people are born with – like a natural artist or singing ability. Don't be hard on yourself if Knowledge Monitoring is not your thing.

The good news is there two very simple ways to compensate for our brain's lack of Knowledge Monitoring.

The first one is FLASHCARDS.

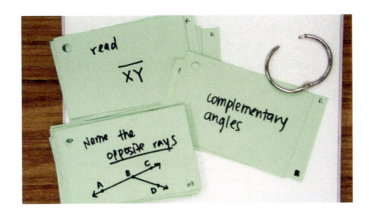

FLASHCARDS

Flashcards are a practical and efficient way to study new things from kindergarten through medical school. They may be the one study method that works for almost everyone. I did an action research study with my Latin I students in 2010. Students who made and used flashcards to study new vocabulary averaged 20 points higher on the Quiz. In fact, students who used flashcards to study NEVER failed a vocabulary quiz. (See data in appendix.)

Here are my suggestions for making flashcards to study:

1) Use index cards because they are precut and uniform.

2) Write the question or vocabulary word on one side of the flashcard card.

3) Write the answer or definition (& any other information you are supposed to know for the test) on the other side of the flashcard.

4) Make your flashcards in a quiet place without distractions. Focus on what you are doing and double check for mistakes. *There is nothing more annoying than learning the wrong answer for the quiz because your flashcard is wrong.*

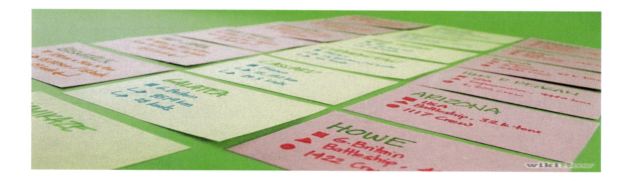

Make your flashcards as early as possible, so you have time to use them to study. Here are my suggestions for using flashcards to study:

1) **Carry the flashcards around with you**. A small ziplock baggie works well for keeping them together. Anytime you have to sit and wait somewhere, you can pull out the flashcards. They will keep you from getting bored and improve your grade.

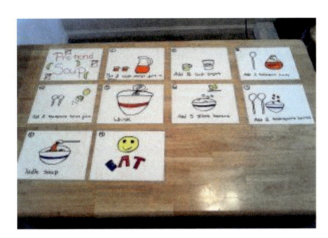

2) As you are studying with flashcards, **make two piles**. One for the words/answers you got correct and one for the ones you missed. The pile of correct flashcards is information you mastered, and you don't need to spend any more time on them. **Spend your study time working on the flashcards you don't know** and keep working until all the flashcards are in the correct pile.

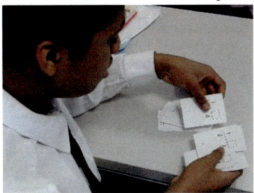

3) Repeat step # 2 three to five times between making the flashcards and taking the quiz/test. **You must use the flashcards to benefit from them**.

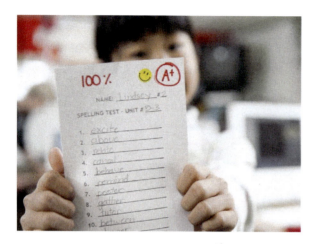

Helpful Hint: Why do flashcards work?

Flashcards work for all Knowledge Monitoring levels. When presented with the question, you can immediately check if your answer is correct by turning the flashcard over. Since you don't stop studying until you have mastered all the flashcards, you don't have to trust your brain's judgement about what it does or doesn't know. In terms of time management, flashcards are easier to carry around than textbooks, notebooks and computers, and can be used anytime, anywhere. THEY ARE THE PERFECT STUDY TOOL.

Reflection

Have you ever used flashcards to study? How long before the quiz did you make the flashcards? How many times did you use the flashcards to study? How did you do on the quiz/test?

___
___
___
___
___

TRY-IT

Try the steps in this book for making and using flashcards to study for your next vocabulary quiz.

How long did you spend using this method to study for quiz? _____

How did you do on the quiz? _____

Now try using flashcards on a different quiz in a different class.

Did the study method work? _____

How did you do on the quiz? _____

Will you use flashcards in the future? Why?

_____
_____
_____
_____
_____
_____

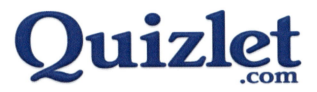

    This is an online tool to make flashcards on a cell phone. Many of my students find it a useful study tool.

The second method that can help you study more effectively whether or not you have good Knowledge Monitoring skills comes from an educational concept called the Testing Effect.

If the first time we "test" to see if we know the answer to the question is on the actual test, then there is no time to fix it when we discover there is something we don't know.

Use metacognition. Be proactive.   If you "test" yourself the day before, then you can be sure you are ready. If you miss questions, there is still time to study what you didn't know.

One way to "test" yourself is create your own quiz/test. Think like the teacher. What do you think they will ask? Write 3-5 questions for yourself, then go do something else for 15-30 minutes.

When you come back, answer the questions you wrote without your notes/textbook and without taking time to study.   Once you have done your best, use your notes/textbook to see what you do and don't know. Like with the flashcards, any answers you get correct, you can stop worrying about and stop studying. Concentrate your time and effort on what you don't know.

The "testing effect" can also be achieved by studying with a partner. The reality is there are a classroom full of students trying to learn the same material you are for the exact same quiz/test. Have you ever heard the expression two heads are better than one? You can call out questions to a classmate and then they can call out questions to you.

I used to give my mother my notes and ask her to quiz me the night before the test. There were several benefits for me in this method.

One – my Mom knew I was studying and trying my best. It made her more understanding if I didn't do so well and even prouder of how hard I worked when I did make a good grade.

Two – if I couldn't watch TV or play video games because I had to study, neither could she. It is said misery loves company. It think the saying should be learning loves company. We are social creatures. No matter what the reason, I will admit I always able to focus and learn more when Mom was helping me.

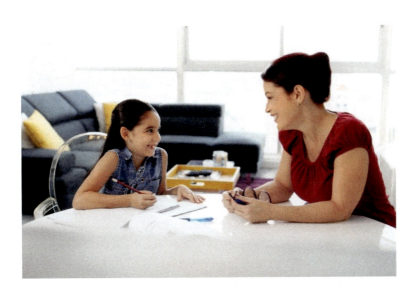

Is There More Than One Way to be Smart?

Dr. Howard Gardner, a professor of Education at Harvard University challenged the idea that intelligence could only be measured by testing or performance on traditional academic assignments. Gardner's Theory of Multiple Intelligences argues that students possess many different talents and mental competences that can influence the types of learning activities that work best for them.

Every brain has a natural ability to learn, understand, and remember new things, yet every brain is different. Some students can easily remember the words of a new song, while other students learn best doing group projects. We all know someone who is gifted in math or who loves to read. There is no one right way to learn. There is more than one type of intelligence. In fact, Gardner argues that there are eight types of intelligence.

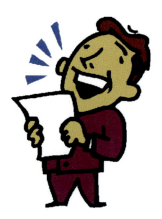

The first type of intelligence is **verbal** (**word smart**). Verbal learners prefer hearing new material and writing assignments. They often report thinking in words and are the friend most likely to correct your spelling on a text. Verbal learners do best on written reports, enjoy the sounds of poetry and drama performed aloud, and are the students who get the most from a teacher's lecture. People with verbal intelligence often become writers, teachers, journalists and lawyers.

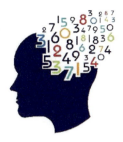

      The second type of intelligence is **logical (math smart)**. Logical learners do well in subjects such as math or physics and are good at solving word problems. They think in patterns and are challenged by mysteries. They are the friend most likely to solve a math problem in their head. Logical learners do well with the scientific method and often devise a strategy when tackling a new problem. Accountants, engineers, statisticians, computer programmers and researchers all tend to be math smart.

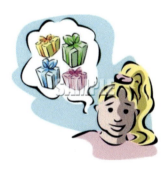

      The third type of intelligence is **visual (art smart)**. Visual learners do best when there is a picture or map involved in the lesson. They tend to think in images and are often excellent artists. They are often good at jigsaw puzzles and photography. They are the friend who can get everything into a car trunk or closet, because they can visualize how everything fits together. Visual learners draw rather than write and design rather than read. Visual learners make good artists, architects, and graphic designers.

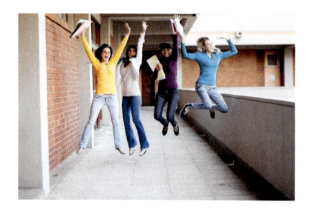

      The fourth type of intelligence is **kinesthetic**. (This is just a fancy word for movement.) Kinesthetic learners are **body smart**. They prefer lessons where they get to use their hands or move around. A kinesthetic learner's favorite subject is probably PE. They think best when they are moving or using manipulatives. They are the friend who is good at sports. Athletes, dancers, and physical therapists all tend to have kinesthetic intelligence.

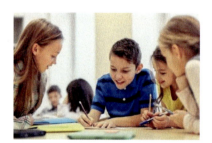

      A fifth type of intelligence is **interpersonal** (**people smart**). As the name suggests interpersonal learners prefer learning in groups or with a partner. These students benefit from interacting with others and often spend as much time thinking about other people and their problems as they do their own issues. An interpersonal learner is that friend who can always tell when you are upset and wants to know how they can help. Therapists, coaches, salesmen, and health care providers all have interpersonal intelligence.

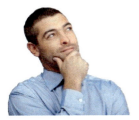

A sixth type of intelligence in intrapersonal (self smart). An intrapersonal learner is a deep thinker. They prefer to work alone rather than in a group. They are self-motivated and often very disciplined. They are the friend most likely to keep a journal or use a habit tracker. People with intrapersonal intelligence are independent learners and the ones who have the easiest time using and improving their metacognition. The fields of philosophy, science, law and theology are all filled with intra personal thinkers.

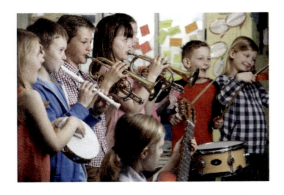

The seventh type of intelligence is **musical (music smart)**. People who are musical learners love to sing, play instruments and listen to music. They take band, orchestra, and choir in school. Musical learners benefit from listening to music while they study. Some even use songs to help them remember lists. If you have a friend who knows the words to every song on the radio, they are probably a musical learner. Some careers for song smart people are musician, singer, choir teacher and DJ.

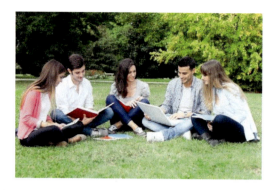

The eighth type of intelligence is **naturalistic** (nature smart). Naturalistic learners enjoy being outside. They love growing plants and taking care of animals. Your friend that is constantly rescuing strays is probably a naturalistic learner. They are sensitive to nature and worried about the environment. They tend to like camping, swimming and hiking. Farmer, animal trainer, veterinarian and horticulturalist are all good careers for people with naturalistic intelligence.

REFLECTION

As you read the descriptions of Gardner's Multiple Intelligences, you probably recognized some of your strengths and preferences. It is normal for people to have characteristics of several different intelligences, although our brains tend to have one to four that are dominate.

To find yours, reread the description of each type of intelligence and decide how well it applies to you.

	This is me EVERYDAY	This is me SOMETIMES	This is me NEVER
VERBAL			✓
LOGICAL			✓
VISUAL			✓
KINESTHETIC		✓	
INTERPERSONAL	✓		
INTRAPERSONAL	✓		
MUSICAL			✓
NATURALIST			✓

Which of Gardner's Multiple Intelligences did you rate as ALWAYS applying to you?

_____

_____

_____

_____

Give examples or experiences that made you suspect these were your dominate intelligences.

_____
_____
_____
_____
_____
_____
_____
_____
_____
_____
_____
_____

TRY-IT

How could you use your dominate intelligences to make learning new things easier? Remember you want to study the way your brain likes to learn.

_____
_____
_____
_____
_____
_____

Here are some suggestions to **maximize learning** for each of
Gardner's Multiple Intelligences.
(There are lines to add your own ideas.)

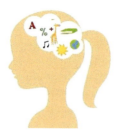

VERBAL

Rewrite important words and definitions.

Record and listen to notes from class.

Read notes and textbook aloud.

_____

_____

LOGICAL

Make a chart to compare and contrast concept you are learning.

Devise a mnemonic to help remember lists.

Rewrite notes as a timeline or Venn diagram.

_use charts_____

_____

VISUAL

Sketch pictures related to new concepts or use color coding and highlighters on your notes.

Picture an image in your mind as you learn new vocabulary words.

Watch videos (with images) about the topic.

_use crash course._____

_____

KINESTHETIC   Try moving while you study.

                       Act out a concept or vocabulary word to help you understand and remember it.

                       Make models to clarify how things work and use manipulatives to solve problems.

                       use Flashcards while moving.

INTERPERSONAL   Discuss what you learn with someone.

                       Have someone quiz you before the test.

                       Work with a study group to prepare for quiz.

                       Help others study

INTRAPERSONAL   Think about and keep a journal of new concepts you are learning and what you think about them.

                       Find a quiet, private place to study.

                       Review graded tests and quizzes. Figure out "why" for any questions you missed.

                       think more about what you need to study.

MUSICAL   Create a song to help you remember concepts and memorize lists.

                       Listen to music while you study. (Something without words is best.)

                       Read notes or main concepts from textbook aloud in a sing-song or rhythmic pattern.

NATURALIST   Try finding a place to study outside.

Listen to nature sounds while studying.

Apply things you learning to real world problems and solutions.

_____

_____

Are you ready for your brain to work smarter?

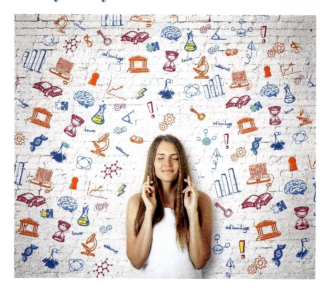

I hope you have found the information in this book useful. ***Remember there is no wrong way to learn. Your brain is unique and the only person who can figure out how it operates is you.***   Never stop trying to make your brain work smarter. Become a life-long learner who can understand and adapt to whatever new knowledge the world decides to throw at you.

I have been on this Earth for a little over a half-century. When I was in school we did not have cell phones, the internet, or Netflix. If I could not think and adapt, I might still be using payphones, encyclopedias and watching reruns on TV.   I like to think my metacognition helped prepare me for the modern world.

Remember - the technology you will be using when you are my age has not been invented yet. To be successful in the future you must be able to learn new things.   You must be able to think about your thinking and understand how your brain learns. Metacognition will be the key to success.

Appendix: KMA Knowledge Monitoring Assessment

If you want to test you knowledge monitoring skill, please follow the directs very carefully. Don't look ahead or "cheat".

Which of these words do you feel you understand the meaning of?
(Can you define it? Can you use it correctly in a sentence? Could you give a synonym?)

	I am confident I know this word.	I am not certain about this word.
amicable	_____	_____
adolescent	_____	_____
celestial	_____	_____
gratelic	_____	_____
loquacious	_____	_____
mortality	_____	_____
paternal	_____	_____
symbiotic	_____	_____
tripod	_____	_____

Now prove you know each word by selecting its synonym or definition.

amicable	friendly	hopeful	pretty	sad
adolescent	crazy	teenager	child	baby
celestial	hard	heavenly	new	careful
loquacious	intelligent	talkative	shy	rude
mortality	death	intelligence	eternal	wicked
paternal	careful	brotherly	mother	fatherly
symbiotic	sensitive	cooperative	harmful	lucky
tripod	one leg	two legs	three legs	four legs

Gratelic not on this list, because it is NOT a word. (It was a control.)

Here are the correct answers.

amicable	**friendly**	hopeful	pretty	sad
adolescent	crazy	**teenager**	child	baby
celestial	hard	**heavenly**	new	careful
loquacious	intelligent	**talkative**	shy	rude
mortality	**death**	intelligence	eternal	wicked
paternal	careful	brotherly	mother	**fatherly**
symbiotic	sensitive	**cooperative**	harmful	lucky
tripod	one leg	two legs	**three legs**	four legs

How to calculate your KMA.   Start with the vocabulary you got correct. Look at page 61. Transfer your answers to this chart columns A & B.   Now look at the words you got wrong. Follow the same procedure in columns C & D.

	CORRECT		WRONG	
	I was confident	I was uncertain	I was confident	I was uncertain
	A	B	C	D
amicable	_____	_____	_____	_____
audacious	_____	_____	_____	_____
circumspect	_____	_____	_____	_____
gratelic		_____	_____	_____
loquacious	_____	_____	_____	_____
nefarious	_____	_____	_____	_____
pragmatic	_____	_____	_____	_____
symbiotic	_____	_____	_____	_____
ubiquitous	_____	_____	_____	_____

A = You are an excellent knowledge monitor and have a strong vocabulary. Trust your judgment when studying.

B = You are a better knowledge monitor than you think you are and have a strong vocabulary. You should try harder to trust your judgment.

C = Your knowledge monitoring skill level is giving you a false sense of confidence. Double check yourself even if you "think" you are right. Try using flashcards to study. They give you immediate feedback and can help improve your knowledge monitoring.

D = The good news is you are an excellent knowledge monitor. The bad news is you know you don't know the vocabulary. All you need is more exposure to words and a little studying.   Trust your judgment and study what you don't know.

Steven Covey's TIME QUADRANTS

	Urgent	Not Urgent
Important	**1 The Procrastinator** *Exam tomorrow *Friend gets injured *Late for work *Project due today *Car breaks down	**2 The Prioritizer** *Planning, Goal setting *Essay due in a week *Exercise *Relationships *Relaxation
Not Important	**3 The "Yes-Man"** *Unimportant phone calls *Interruptions *Other people's small problems *Peer Pressure	**4 The Slacker** *Too much tv *Endless phone calls *Excessive computer games *Mall marathons *Time wasters

As this visual from Covey's book shows, I didn't do the quadrants in the same order he did. He explains the types of time management in respect to an X/Y axis with important/not important and urgent/not urgent. It is part of Habit #3 – putting first things first. I highly recommend you read Steven Covey's *7 Habits of Highly Effective Teens.*

The Origins of Metacognition

The term metacognition began with an American developmental psychologist named John H. Flavell. Educational researchers had been studying smart students (the ones that were more successful in school) and trying to define what characteristics and skills made them smarter than their peers. Flavell and others found that smart students often did better than their peers in multiple subjects. How could they be better in math, science, reading, and history? They couldn't all have stronger background knowledge or more interest in the subject. Some other factor had to be at work.

It turned out that most smart students did have one thing in common. They were all good at learning new things. They could explain how they learned, learn from their mistakes, and knew what study methods worked best for them. They thought about learning. Researchers had discovered what made some students smarter than others and thus was born the science of metacognition.

Flavell defined metacognition as knowledge about and control of one's thinking. Metacognition is a process. For example, a person who is engaging in metacognition notices that they are having more trouble learning Biology than learning English. They think about the similarities and differences in their approaches to learning those two subjects and decide what factors might be making Biology harder. A metacognitive thinker then systematically experiments with new ways to study Biology. They don't stop trying out new ways to learn until they find the ones that help them understand and remember Biology most effectively.

Metacognition can be as important to the learning process as the content of the subject. Novice learners spend all of their time and effort studying with little planning or reflection. Sometimes they are successful and sometimes they are not. To be a metacognitive learner, students think about and plan for studying. How else can they be sure they spend enough time and study the right material. After they get back their grade on the quiz or test, a metacognitive learner will reflect on how well their studying worked and how it might be improved in the future. To truly use and improve metacognition a student must not just understand how their brain works but continually monitor and adjust their efforts to maximize learning.

Flashcard Data from Andrea Stehle's 2010 action research study on Latin Vocabulary

Procedure: Thirty-three students were given the option of making and using flashcards to study for the vocabulary quiz at the end of each stage in the Cambridge Latin Course. I looked at grades on multiple quizzes over the course of an entire semester.

*This is the percentage of the students who made and used flashcards to study. Since it was a voluntary study method, it changed with each quiz.

	Average Grade on Vocab Quiz
Stage 15 with flashcards (40%)*	83
Stage 15	79
Stage 16 with flashcards (49%)	88
Stage 16	70
Stage 17 with flashcards (54%)	90
Stage 17	62
Stage 18 with flashcards (61%)	93
Stage 18	60
Stage 19 with flashcards (66%)	95
Stage 19	63
OVERALL Average with flashcards	90
OVERALL Average	67

By the end of the study there was a 23 point gap in the average grade on the vocabulary quiz between students who used flashcards to study and those who did not. I was disappointed that there was a small percentage of students (8%) who never made flashcards for any stage vocabulary and never passed any of the quizzes. Their lack of effort brought down the "non-flashcard" average.

The upward trend of students using flashcards to study and the increasing average on the "flashcard" students' vocabulary quiz grade was a natural occurrence during the study. Because I shared the flashcard vs non-flashcard average after each quiz, more and more students decided to "try" using flashcards to study. Student wanted to do better on the vocabulary quizzes and saw how others were doing it. **Success inspired more success**.

I noticed the grade improvement for students who had been struggling to pass vocabulary quizzes in the past was even more significant. It allowed most of them to move from failing or barely passing to consistently making 80 or better.

During this study, every student who made and used flashcards to study (THE METHOD SUGGESTED IN THIS BOOK p. 46) passed the vocabulary quiz.

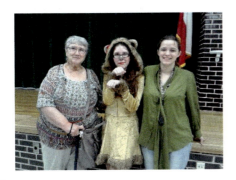

Gratias tibi ago

     I want to thank my students at BASIS who suggested I write this book after my study skills workshop. It was a good idea. It was meant to be. I only took 3 months to write this book. That is MUCH FASTER than any book in my sci-fi mythology series, Gods of Arcadia.

     I must acknowledge the woman who has read and critiqued every word I have ever written from school assignments when I was little, through my poetry & short story phase, and finally my first novel, Daughter of Athena. I love you, Mom. Thank you for supporting me no matter what I want to try.

     My three beautiful daughters, Monica, Amanda and Linda, have inspired me to try to be a better Mom and a better person who sees the potential in everyone and tries to help others follow their dreams. I am a better Student Success Advisor because I try to give students the same opportunities I would want for my own children.

     Finally, I would like to thank Harold Maldonado and Michelle Craig who took a chance on me. Being the Student Success Advisor at Stevens High School was one of the best parts of my thirty-year career. This book was so easy to write, because you let me pursue my passion to make a difference. I never knew how much I learned until today.

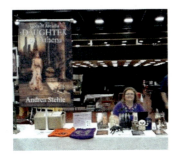
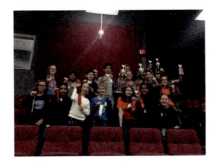

You can contact me at **magistrastehle@yahoo.com** .

Made in the USA
Columbia, SC
28 July 2019